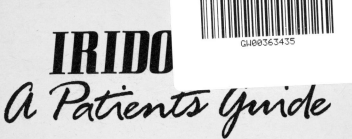

IRIDO

A Patients Guide

An introduction to iridology, the
concept of diagnosis based on
individual iris patterns.

IRIDOLOGY
A Patient's Guide

James and Sheelagh Colton

THORSONS PUBLISHING GROUP
Wellingborough, Northamptonshire

First published 1988

© James and Sheelagh Colton 1988

British Library Cataloguing in Publication Data

Colton, James
Iridology: a patients guide.
1. Iris (Eye) — Examination   2. Ocular
manifestations of general diseases
I. Title   II. Colton, Sheelagh
616.07'54   RC73.5

ISBN 0-7225-1516-2

Published by Thorsons Publishers Limited,
Wellingborough, Northamptonshire, NN8 2RQ, England

Printed in Great Britain by Richard Clay Limited,
Bungay, Suffolk

1 3 5 7 9 10 8 6 4 2

Contents

Foreword

We have long had a need of a precise and practical introduction to iridology. James and Sheelagh Colton's book *Iridology, A Patient's Guide*, fulfils that need. It goes further; it shows that accurate iris diagnosis within a medical context is more than just a sum of its markings, structures, pigmentation, and colour variation. Done precisely and intelligently it bears witness to human totality and that totality speaks not just of the present or the past but of the potential for health or illness in the future. How many other diagnostic methods can do this?

Iris analysis offers information that is simply not available through conventional laboratory tests and interpretations of a patient's symptoms. These may show that something is wrong but they seldom reveal which organ is affected. Iridology does this effectively, efficiently and reliably *without* requiring exploratory surgery, tissue biopsies, injections of dyes or chemicals to make organs appear distinct on X-Ray, or other uncomfortable and expensive diagnostic aids. Iridology is painless, safe, non-invasive and above all accurate provided it is done by a competent, well-trained and experienced practitioner.

James and Sheelagh satisfy all these categories. They both have an extraordinary combination of in-depth knowledge and highly developed intuition and inventiveness. Which does not mean they give any truck to a clairvoyant or mystical approach to iridology, and sadly there is some of that going around, debasing iridology.

A good iris diagnostician will first take a detailed case history. I give my patients a seven-page questionnaire to fill out before they see me and many of them are surprised that I want information that their own doctors have never asked for. He will then consider the acute event that has brought the patient to see him. Most of my patients come and see me in the throes of a crisis. Only one or two per cent of the thousands of patients I have worked with to date actually come in for a general preventative check up. Sadly, most wait until a break down occurs before asking for help. A good iris diagnostician will then assess the relevance of iris diagnosis to the particular case he is working with. The causes of osteoarthritis are manifold though the results may be approximately the same.

I never attempt to take care of any disease. Instead I take care of the person and iridology in its totality shows me the way. That is prevention at its best. I am a fervent believer in 'more educating, less medicating'. Would I were given the chance to practise it fully! Patients would tease me about the amount my photocopier is used and wonder when I find the time to write books, do television programmes and lecture. But all this 'spreading the gospel', as I call it, is the pre-requisite of a good practitioner. Teach patients how to make tissue changes during the preclinical stage of any illness and you're no longer fighting a losing battle with the symptoms but building very real and enduring well-being. Best of all, you are giving power back to the patient, and when a distressing number of mine have been mauled about and finally rejected by a system which might with some justification be called the National *Illness* Service this is victory indeed. Such an outlook means commitment from the patient. I am occasionally tempted to put a sign up outside my consulting room saying, 'You may be looking for a good doctor, but I am looking for good patients!'. But generally when we meet half way the effort is incredibly rewarding.

James and Sheelagh both share that delight. James is well trained in the German method of natural medicine: Sheelagh in nutrition. Wherever possible they work together, share patients, share notes and lecture together. They are a constant source of inspiration to each other and they have shared their vast experience in iridology selflessly and unstintingly. Firstly by founding the National Council and Register of Iridology (N.C.R.Ir.) in 1983, and secondly by setting up the Bournemouth Free Iridology Clinic where patients can come for free iris evaluation. This has enabled them to expand their already considerable photographic slide library with a further twelve thousand sets of iris slides. This has led to the development of the British Iris Chart, published in 1986.

I am privileged to have started as one of their students and become one of their friends. They have supported my studies and sustained my enthusiasm for and commitment to iridology. I hope that their introduction to iridology will be widely read and open mindedly investigated and that it will prove a blessing to many.

KITTY CAMPION

Introduction

Imagine being ill and not knowing *why*. Imagine having a tremendous thirst, with dizzy spells or periods of extreme tiredness and weakness with odd cravings only to be told 'There is nothing wrong with you.' Modern technical diagnosis in its science has entered realms beyond our wildest dreams. Left in the wake of these advancements are many people who find little or no help when the hospital tests prove negative.

Forty years ago Dr A. Clarke-Kennedy, who was Physician to the London Hospital and Dean of the Medical School, was probably one of the first to show disapproval of the system that was beginning to demoralize patients. He believed that, because of bureaucratic organization, the established medical profession was in danger of training their doctors in highly specialist categories. This, he believed, had an adverse effect on patients; they had a right to know why they were ill. Training, which is based solely on hard facts, does not develop intuition, understanding, love or compassion. Laboratory tests and impersonal equipment were fast replacing the close personal contact between doctor and patient, and there was less chance that account would be taken of *why* health problems had arisen. For instance, a patient with a pancreas that had begun to hypofunction may perhaps be mourning the recent loss of a loved one and, as a consequence, be under a great deal of stress – a condition which is known to affect the pancreas. The laboratory tests would suggest diabetes, so the immediate conclusion would be that the patient had become diabetic. But, it could be that when stress levels had reduced, the patient's pancreas would return to normal functioning.

Today we are all witnesses to the progression of impersonal medicine.

The iridologist endeavours to give a total account of the patient's symptoms and, by studying the iris, he will see the patient in his total complexity.

This benefits the patient in many ways. For example, let's take a person who suffers with migraine headaches. The cause of migraine could be (1) spinal lesion, (2) liver congestion, or (3) food allergy. The iridologist has at his disposal techniques for identifying the root cause making treatment easy to apply.

Iridology not only benefits the sick but also the well. Many of our patients come to us for prevention of disease for, in evaluating wellness, the iris reveals genetic factors which must be taken into account as well as exogenous factors.

In studying the iris, the coloured part of the eye, the iridologist views a totally unique structure. Each person has an individual iris pattern in the same way that each person has individual fingerprints. However, similarities in iris patterns exist and have been recorded by iridologists for hundreds of years. In the United Kingdom the National Council and Register of Iridologists has joined other world-wide organizations in this research; they also provide training courses.

This book outlines the way in which Iridology was rediscovered in the 1800s by Ignaz von Peczely, and the reason why he devoted his life to studying the iris. Illustrations and explanations of some of the iris markings are given along with treatments. The book dispels myths and misconceptions and gives a clear account of the possible limitations of Iris Diagnosis.

This book is intended for two kinds of people: those with a

health problem they wish to improve and those who are healthy and wish to stay that way. Treatments are purely academic; there are herbal alternatives to aspirin, and there is an alternative treatment for spinal problems, but there is no alternative for a correct diagnosis. It is the diagnosis which has to be right. Many prospective patients will not be surprised to know that many established practitioners of alternative/complementary medicine combine the diagnostic benefits of iridology with those of their own particular therapy: homoeopathy, acupuncture, herbalism or whatever. Indeed, in Germany, most homoeopathic doctors have iridology as part of their training curriculum. The British patient will find that one iridologist will be more experienced in diagnosing a broader range of illness and disease than another.

The training one iridologist receives from one school is not necessarily the same as that given from another school. Therefore, once you have made the decision to visit an iridologist, it is of vital importance that you have confidence in his or her diagnostic abilities. This book will make it easier for you to choose the right practitioner. The sort of guidelines to follow (which will be discussed later on in Chapter 10) are:

1. How long has he been in practice?
2. Does he work by a code of ethics?
3. Is he registered with his school?
4. How long was his training (18 months minimum)?
5. Did his training include anatomy and physiology?

In Great Britain there are no laws (yet) governing the practice of alternative and complementary therapies.

Iridology is neither complementary nor alternative. It is part of a whole branch of medicine that is established to determine the patient's state of health. In principle, it is no different to an X-ray, ultrasound scan or magnetic scanning system. However, it definitely is not involved with seeing into a person's soul nor will it tell you what the future holds.

In our own experience there are very few doctors who would refuse to work with an iridologist for the benefit of the patient. This is why such a high training standard must be obtained.

James and Sheelagh Colton

1

The Beginning

One crisp winter's morning a boy named Ignaz fought with an owl he had tried to capture; the bird had dug its claws into his arm and was fighting for its life. Ignaz was filled with panic and desperately tried to free himself from the bird's sharp talons. In the confusion that followed the bird's leg was broken. The boy wrapped the bird in his coat and swiftly took it home, for he felt compelled to heal it. As he bandaged the broken leg their gazes met and Ignaz at once noticed a small black dot in the bird's eye. The next morning the dot had become a black line running from the pupil to the edge of the iris.

After its leg healed, the owl stayed with Ignaz even though it was free to fly away. Several months later, Ignaz noticed that the black line began to disappear from the bird's eye until all the remained was a white line. This encounter with the owl led Ignaz to care for and study other animals and was to be the beginning of modern iris diagnosis.

Later, Ignaz Peczely became a brilliant student graduating in engineering, but the impression and feeling he had experienced with healing the owl never left him. He went on to study medicine in Budapest and graduated there.

His patients provided him with ample opportunity to study the iris and from these studies he located specific organ zones in the iris. His location of the stomach zone was so accurate (he went to Vienna to confirm this with Professor Billroth in 1881), its position in the iris map remains the same today.

Other Iris Researchers

In Sweden, around the same time, Pastor Nils Liljequist stumbled on the connection of various colours and pigmentations in the iris with disease. After being treated with large doses of quinine for a major illness, he discovered, to his horror, that his eyes had changed from blue to a yellow/green colour. Liljequist eventually met Peczely in Budapest and they became lifelong friends. Their pioneering instincts created the beginnings of iris topography. Others were soon to follow: Pastor Felke who gave up his ministry in 1912 to devote himself to healing the sick. He was among the greatest therapists of his time and his fame as an iridologist spread far beyond the borders of his native Germany. The basis of Felke's work lies in his belief that the iris dictates the prescription.

Students of Felke

Students of Felke continued his research into iris diagnosis. Magdalene Madaus (1857–1925) contributed a great deal to this science and she herself acquired many followers. She was responsible for founding the Association of Iridologists and, in 1915, published a textbook on ocular diagnosis. Her daughter, Mrs Eva Flink (1886–1959), continued her mother's work and edited the third edition of her mother's book *Ocular Diagnosis*. She was also the editor of *Iris Correspondence* for many years. Another student of Felke's was Alfred Maubach (1893–1954) who was a pupil of outstanding quality and developed general photography of the iris. He was one of the first iridologists to use a corneal microscope and in 1952 wrote *Constitutional Aspects of Ocular Diagnosis* and became the co-founder of the International Research Circle for Ocular Diagnosis.

Wilhelm Poullie also became enthusiastic about iris diagnosis when he was cured from a serious internal disease by Felke. He became an iris diagnostician and he furthered the development of iris photography. Wilhelm Zahres (1877–

1954) was also cured by Felke from a serious illness and became probably one of the most talented of all Felke's students. In 1903 he set up as a naturopath and was always active in the promotion of iris diagnosis. In 1927 he founded a sanatorium where iris diagnosis was used extensively in healing the sick.

The great iris diagnostician Rudolf Schnabel (1882–1952) contributed much to the advancement of iridology. Although he originally trained as a teacher he could not ignore the pull of natural medicine. At the age of 22 he cured a young child who had previously been unable to walk. In 1915 he wrote an article *The Eyes as a Mirror of Health* which resulted in his being expelled from university. He then moved to Munich and founded a laboratory for Applied Ophthalmologic-Physiological and Diagnostic Auxiliary Sciences. His success grew and earned him universal fame as well as several honorary medical degrees. He wrote many textbooks including *Symptoms of the Outer Eye in Diseases of the Organism*. Unfortunately, his half dozen or so books were published in German and have not yet been translated into English. No doubt they soon will be as iridology is increasing in popularity amongst serious iris researchers. This list of Felke's students and graduates is not intended to be complete; there are many others who would be worthy of mentioning had space permitted.

Modern Researchers
Recent contributors include Josef Angerer of Munich whose works we have translated into English for our own research purposes, Dr Bernard Jensen of Escondido, USA, Dr Bruce Halstead of Colton, California, USA, Josef Deck of Germany and Dr Vanier of France. In England there is a small group of iris researchers. They include John Morley of London, David Bartlett of Bath, Kitty Campion of Stoke-on-Trent and ourselves. Again, this list is not intended to be complete.

Because iris signs are empirical and because, as Schnabel

taught, those who believe or would like to believe that learning iridology can be achieved in a few weeks or even days are mistaken and do a disservice to a good cause, iridology, like radiology, takes many years to learn. The iridologist has to develop his intuition, he has to understand many aspects of health and disease, and his training has to enable him to explain medical conditions to his patient. However, the true scientific evaluation of iris diagnosis will go on, for the benefits it provides cannot be ignored.

Empirical Observations

Iris diagnosis is based on empirical observations over many hundreds of years. There have been attempts, mainly in Germany, to evaluate iris diagnosis scientifically but these attempts have been rejected as being undesirable to present diagnostic procedures. Can we assume that this is because there is little or no commercial incentive in pursuing this research further? In Russia iris research is funded by the State and some amazing results have been published. What is right and good cannot be suppressed for long and, in today's environment of alternative medicine, the public are demanding to be seen and treated as individuals. The whole concept of iris diagnosis is based on individual genetic patterns.

New approaches to diagnosing gives the patient the choice of treatments. The opportunity of choosing what type of treatment you receive will not only give you, the patient, the psychological benefits of being responsible for your own body but, more importantly, allow you to take an active part in your recovery.

If a patient is seen to have genetic weakness of the heart, the iridologist can present them with the choice of taking steps to strengthen their heart by means of nutrition, life-style, supplements and so on. If, on the other hand, the patient has had a heart attack then the iridologist will recommend whatever care is appropriate. The iridologist endeavours always to keep a balance between prevention and action, still allowing the patient the right to choose.

Case History

Mrs B. originally came to see if all was well. Although her husband pooh-poohed the idea, she felt instinctively there was something wrong. She was an attractive woman of 38 years old with three teenage children, and had been feeling extra tired lately. While examing her iris we saw clearly an iris marking known as a radial platt in her cervix/womb area. This was surrounded by what iridologists call peppercorn markings and indicated chronic irritation to the area concerned. A change in the cell structure, possibly pre-cancer of her cervix/womb was indicated. She confirmed that she was experiencing unusually irregular periods but she reported no pain or discomfort. We suggested that there was no time to lose in having a cervical smear test. This proved positive. Her husband still did not see that there was anything to make such a fuss about. We spent a couple of hours reassuring her and together we worked out a plan to ensure her best health. This was before she had the cauterization operation advised by her doctors and to which she readily agreed. Our action was a special vitamin and mineral formula, a diet based on very high quality foods, and relaxation exercises. Two months later she felt much better and fit enough to have the operation. This was successful and, to date, some four years later, she has had no further problems.

Sometimes it is possible that the patient does not or cannot, for one reason or another, take responsibility for a problem that faces them. The severity of the problem may be too difficult to cope with, or the very nature of the illness prevents the patient from taking control for himself. Sometimes an over-emotional state can bring about the illness, such as anorexia nervosa in which the patient loses the desire to eat. However, if an emotionally-based disease is detected early enough and subsequently treated, it will not take its full course.

The iridologist has a clear understanding of what is physical and what is imaginary. He is often able to stabilize those who find emotional problems hard to cope with and, by his very nature, can decide the best way to avoid an illness developing because of stress factors. He knows that the conflict between the brain and the body in terms of the origin of a disease must be resolved with the aid of a psychologist.

We have often wondered how many national work days would be saved if sick notes were obtained only from iridologists. We remember talking about the problem of staff absences to the junior houseman of a large hospital. He asked us how an iridologist would determine if someone was shamming unconsciousness. 'We do not know' we said. He replied that it was simple. 'Those that are unconscious have their eyes half open while those who are shamming have them tightly closed.'

2

What is Iris Diagnosis?
Why the Iris Reveals Bodily Conditions

When a patient has his health and fitness analyzed by iris diagnosis, it is possible to recognize the root cause of a particular disease. We know that the cause of natural death is indicated by markings in the iris; a person who dies of a heart attack will almost certainly have a marking in the heart zone of his iris. This phenomenon has been studied, sometimes at post-mortem, over the last fifty years. Premature death, say by a road traffic accident or a toxic dose of some dangerous chemical, is, of course, not recorded by the iris because it is not a natural death for the individual. Post-mortem findings could reveal what the natural death would have been had the person lived out his natural life-span.

Having a diagnosis and discussing a course for preventing future disease at a time when a patient appears completely healthy and symptom-free appears to make the orthodox medical world uneasy. This is probably because they are more geared to dealing with the disease itself and do not accept readily the idea of preventing that disease. Diabetes is a very good example of this kind of thinking. A diabetic patient can be treated with insulin, whereas a milder case may be treated by strict diet control. However, the idea that there is a state of pre-diabetes is a litle more difficult to comprehend but, from examining the iris, the iridologist may suspect diabetes will become a problem at a later stage of life. No other form of diagnosis could determine future health trends in this way.

However, disarming it may be, the fact remains that the iridologist usually can determine the health and disease patterns of individuals. This is why we believe it is so necessary for the medical establishment to allow iridologists the chance to work with doctors in a hospital environment, to prove and extend their case.

How it Works
There is no organ as minutely complex as the eye. It has millions of electrical connections and it can handle one and a half million messages – all at the same time. The eye contributes about 80 per cent of all the knowledge and experience gathered by the body. Compared to a tiny television camera, the eye is far more complex. The visible part of the eye consists of:

1. The pupil, the black centre, an adjustable gateway for light. In poor light the pupil dilates to allow extra light into the eye.
2. The iris, the coloured part of the eye and the part we are mainly concerned with.
3. The sclera – the white of the eye.

The Importance of Reflexes
The systems responsible for producing body fluids and chemicals allow information to be passed from one organ to the next, and from one system to another. The whole system can function only on the basis of being able to pass on chemical messages. Incoming data has to be received, absorbed and passed on. Decisions have to be made and new impulses sent out. Chemical and electrical activity within the organism is constantly trying to overcome disorders of health by applying the same criteria. This is often quite inadequate, producing the same reaction to a variety of irritations. This is the diathesis of the condition.

One such condition is the cold virus. The reaction it causes to the body is the same, or very similar, each time; catarrh, sore throat, headache and so on. This, in turn, causes a disturbance of the sensitive endocrine system to rid the body of toxins stored in the tissues. Many of these systems work under reflex actions – an automatic or involuntary activity brought about by relatively simple nerve circuits; we do not need to think about reflex actions or even be conscious. We become wide awake when a sudden, unusual noise interferes with normal sleep, when the finger is pricked with a sharp pin the stimuli bring about a very speedy withdrawal of the finger before the brain has had time to send a message to the muscle involved. It is these reflexes which are carried by the sympathetic nervous system to the iris. The subsequent markings are known as reflex markings and differ from genetic markings of disposition. The former have been noted to change, unlike those markings of genetic disposition.

It is well documented that the iris receives complex nerve connections. Dr. W. Lang in his work *Anatomical and Physiological Principles of Ocular Diagnosis* (1946) demonstrates the presence of nervous connections from the organs, via the spinal cord and the ciliospinal centre, to the iris. Before entering the iris, nerve impulses travel the length of the spinal cord and they do this in a highly organized way. It has been found that nerves entering the lower part, and then leading to the upper part of the spinal cord, are so designed that within the spinal cord itself bundles of nerve fibres are laid down one on top of the other in a strict order, reaching into the ciliospinal centre. Nerve impulses here are transmitted to the iris via switch-over points.

Research

Recent research has discovered small receptors in the eyes of animals that have the ability to change their skin colour like chameleons, the long-tongued lizards which change colour

according to their surroundings. This automatic reflex action
has amazed mankind for centuries. Perhaps future research
will reveal the presence of similar receptors in the human eye,
maybe not for changing our skin colour, but to analyze our
surroundings. This could be why some people instinctively do
not like certain landscapes. We know people who prefer the
unending flatness of Lincolnshire while others prefer to gaze
down at undulating hills. These receptors, if present, could
explain why some people find it difficult to settle when they
move from one area to another. It is also possible that such
receptors may react in a similar way to how our brain reacts to
smell. Recent research by Steve van Toller, of the Olfaction
Research Group at Warwick University, UK, has shown that
odour inhalation produces an immediate response in the
brain. He claims there are close links between olfaction (sense
of smell), emotion and cognition. This is the basis of
aromatherapy, the massage treatment which uses essential
oils.

Our own studies have linked the diagnosis of intestinal
overgrowth of *candida albicans* with the iris. Because candida is
a part of the *normal* flora of the bowel and lives, to a limited
extent, in all of us, it shows no marking within the iris. The iris
will record only what is *abnormal*. Under normal, healthy conditions the 'friendly' bacteria keep this unfriendly resident at
bay and prevent candida from becoming a problem. When
something occurs to upset the normal ratio of 'good' to 'bad'
bacteria, this is the chance candida waits for and it bursts forth
and multiplies. The iris is slightly behind what is happening
inside the body and the very early stages of this infestation do
not make their mark in the iris. As yet, we have not yet
recognized any iris marking relating to this early infestation
(though we are able to scan early iris pictures of the patients
who have, some years later, developed candidiasis). As the
yeast thrives and multiplies in its ideal environment (warm,
moist and dark) the iris begins to take on a peculiar colour.

The area directly next to the pupil becomes darker and muddy-looking. In a blue iris, this zone, the digestive tract, becomes quite dark and easily identified even with the naked eye. In a brown iris, it is still possible to detect the even darker, almost grey/brown discolouration, but it is made easier with magnification. In the 1970s the Japanese mycologist, Kazuo Iwata, found that as the yeast dies it splits open, releasing toxins that can weaken the immune system. It is these toxins that we can now identify as a specific pigmentation in the iris. Candida is responsible for many unpleasant symptoms:

1. Feeling tired most of the time.
2. Intestinal gas/abnormal bloating.
3. Recurrent irritability.
4. Halitosis (bad breath).
5. Feeling light-headed or dizzy.
6. Difficulty in concentrating.
7. Loss of sexual desire.
8. Anxiety attacks.
9. Depression.
10. Craving for sugar, bread, beer or other alcoholic drinks.
11. Food allergies.

Many practitioners are becoming interested and aware of the effects of an overgrowth of candida. Dr Harry Howell runs Britain's first centre for the treatment and study of *candida albicans* and, having studied our work on the subject, he now incorporates iris diagnosis to help him detect the overgrowth syndrome.

3

The Consultation

Many of my patients have said that going to an iridologist is a unique experience. At the consultation the iridologist will discuss with you the many aspects of your individual health, some of which may be a little unexpected. Past events, such as old injuries or illnesses from long ago, often become the topic of conversation. Although one or two people may be a little nervous at first, the iridologist has the skill to relax you. Iridologists conduct their consultations in a variety of ways. This is important and proves most valuable because it allows flexibility when interviewing the patient. As everyone is different, with different worries and personalities, it is necessary to alter the approach slightly to suit the needs of the patient.

The first consideration in a diagnosis from the iris is the colour. Brown, blue and grey are the only 'true' iris colours; any other colour, such as green and hazel, are not really there at all and are therefore 'false' colours. When you look closely, through a magnifying glass, at an apparently hazel-coloured eye, you will find it is really blue with patches of brown on top. The illusion of the green eye is created by yellow pigmentation on a blue iris; sometimes this can indicate liver or gallbladder troubles. It is the colour which gives the iridologist the first insight to the patient's constitution type.

Next, the structure of the iris is considered. Every person has their own structure or pattern to the iris. This structure will reveal organ markings, such as lacunas, honeycombs and tulips. Then the iris examiner begins to study each marking individually, assessing the severity and position. The patient is asked various questions to ascertain the condition of the organ in question.

You may find the iridologist spends some time in determining the significance of the organ marking. He will need to know whether the marking indicates a latent condition or if the condition has become active. A marking in the kidney zone is more significant if the patient is experiencing dull pain in the lower back. You can see why it is so necessary for the iridologist to have studied in depth physical symptoms, aetiology and prognosis.

The Lupe Reading

Initially the iris is examined with a magnifying glass which enlarges the appearance of the iris about six times. An ordinary penlight is used to illuminate the iris – this does not hurt the eye in any way. The iris is studied carefully against an iris chart and all markings and pigmentations systematically recorded. The amount of light cast onto the iris is kept to a minimum especially if the eyes are sensitive to light. When a young child is to be examined we find it helpful, to both the child and ourselves, if the child sits comfortably on his mother's knee. This encourages the child to keep quite still and his gaze constant, for the patient's eyes must be still so that the practitioner can observe. Talking quietly to a young patient and reassuring him usually works well.

Next, the zones marked in the iris are discussed with the patient. It is now that the iridologist's skill in accumulating the facts about your symptoms, both past and present, comes to light. Details of your family history may be recorded. If the iridologist suspects a blood sugar imbalance, he may ask if anyone in your family has diabetes. This gives him a clearer picture as to the severity of the iris sign he has just seen. Now is also the time when details are taken of any surgery and drug administration. If the patient has undergone surgery of any kind, there can no longer be a relevant record of the organ in the iris. If a patient has had their appendix removed, the iridologist can see only the condition that it *was* in when it was still in the body. So, even twenty years later, the iris may still record an inflamed appendix zone but it has little relevance to the patient's health problem today.

Some drugs may alter the colour of the iris and, if the colour of the iris is abnormal, the iridologist needs to know whether it is caused by drugs, or whether there is an underlying bodily process which is causing the iris to be discoloured.

Later, the iridologist will take a photograph, using a specially adapted camera enabling him to take a close-up picture of your iris. By projecting the 35mm slide onto a screen, your iris picture can be enlarged even further – to about 20 times its normal size. Photographing the iris has another advantage; it provides an ideal record of the health and condition of the patient and is invaluable for future reference. The slide can then be compared with a new photograph at a later date, providing it is taken under the same strict conditions of light, camera settings and so on. Slightly over-expose a picture and the iris appears lighter in colour and can give the illusion that the patient's condition has improved. On the other hand, under-exposing the picture will make it slightly darker, giving the illusion that the condition is worse!

Some iridologists use a stereo microscope which allows a very good enlargement of the iris. This makes it possible to see a deeper underlying pathological condition (if there is one) at the time of the consultation. The only drawback to using a stereo microscope is that with any magnification over 12 times the original size, the iridologist loses the view of the whole iris, and thus the whole person. However, these microscopes are gaining favour and we are sure that before long, nearly every iridologist will be using one.

Other Tests

Most people will be used to their family doctor examining them and perhaps applying one or two physical tests such as taking your blood pressure or looking at your throat. The iridologist goes one step further. He may decide to apply four or five tests during the consultation to help determine whether the iris marking is now in its active stage. If you show a positive result to one or more of the tests, the iridologist will probably recommend a specific course of treatment and a further consultation at a later date.

If the iris indicates a disturbance in the adrenals, the iridologist may assess your adrenal efficiency by applying this simple test. After resting for five minutes the blood pressure is taken while lying down. You are then asked to stand up and the blood pressure is immediately taken again. If the second reading is not at least five points higher than the first, it confirms under-functioning of the adrenals. Disturbances seen in the thyroid zone of the iris can also be confirmed by a simple physical test. It requires the patient to take their underarm temperature on waking for three consecutive mornings. An average temperature is obtained and should be recorded. If the result is below 36.5° C (97.8° F) the thyroid is underactive; if above 36.8° C (98.2° F) the thyroid is overactive. Although Dr Stephen Langer M. D. claims that in rare instances the temperature does not rise as high as normal. Large doses of vitamin C may also inhibit the test. Therefore we feel that any such test should be medically supervised.

If the iris displays severe disturbances in the gastrointestinal zone the Gastro Test may be applied. While lying down, the patient is asked to swallow a soluble capsule containing a specially prepared, fine, nylon thread. One end of the thread is attached with sticking plaster to the cheek edge of the mouth, enabling the thread to unwind, down the gut and into the stomach as it is swallowed. After ten minutes the thread is gently retrieved and compared closely to a Ph chart to determine acid/alkaline activity in different areas of the upper digestive tract. Although this test may sound a little drastic, it is quite painless. The Gastro Test can help determine bleeding in the stomach, bleeding in the oesophagus, pernicious anaemia and achlorhydria (lack of stomach acid).

When the iris displays a marking in the heart zone, there are two simple tests that could be applied to determine the organ condition. The first is the Step-Up Test.

The Step-Up Test
1. Your pulse is taken after ten minutes of quiet rest. The result might be 80 bpm (heart beats per minute) for example.

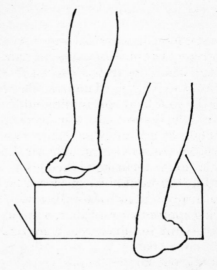

Figure 3.1   The step-up test

2. You are then asked to step up and down a step (or sturdy wooden box, or similar), which is approximately 30 cm high, at the rate of one step per second. This is repeated 75 times.
3. On completion, your pulse is taken immediately. Your pulse will rise, to 100 bpm, for example.
4. You will now take rest for 5 minutes and then your pulse is taken again. It should return to the original figure, i.e. 80 bpm.

If you experience pain in the chest, the iridologist will stop the test. If your pulse rate stays higher than it was when the test was started, it could confirm the iris marking and medical attention will be needed. If your pulse rate stays the same during the test, it could indicate heart/nerve problems needing medical attention. The physically weak may not be able to complete this test. In this case, medical attention is needed for the reason of weakness.

Blood Pressure
The second test is more familiar and often applied to establish early warning signs of trouble. Most people have, at some time or another, had their blood pressure taken. Half of all hypertensives are unaware of their condition. This fact alone is a good reason why your blood pressure should be checked frequently. All iridologists will take your blood pressure as an integral part of the consultation but, in the presence of a heart marking, it will be viewed more carefully. He will not leave you in any doubt as to the meaning of the figures. For example, a reading of 185/120 would be considered high and, in the presence of a corresponding iris marking, would need gentle treatment using appropriate remedies to suit individual cases to lower the pressure in the veins and arteries.

The Finger Wrinkle Test
The purpose of this test is to establish healthy reactions of the

sympathetic nervous system. Along with the antagonistic re-actions of the parasympathetic nervous system, it helps to control the heart rate, blood pressure, breathing, pupil size, digestion, urination, sweating, the tears of crying, stuffiness of the nose, some sexual reactions, wrinkling of the skin and yawning. One hand is placed in a bowl of warm water for at least half an hour. Part of the sympathetic nervous system reacts and wrinkles the skin of the fingers. If your fingers do not wrinkle, it can indicate a nerve infection, heart and/or artery disease, anaemia, or hormone imbalance such as diabetes. Alcohol and drug abuse may also interfere with normal sympathetic nervous system activity.

These tests are often of vital importance for they not only help the patient to know and understand the condition of his own body but also give the doctor access to familiar test results should the patient require further hospital investigations. Usually we find the family doctor will be happy to refer the patient to the hospital specialist whenever necessary.

As previously stated, the body usually responds in the same way to a particular illness which we may call the symptoms of disease. There are about six hundred documented symptoms and it is important that the iridologist is familar with the majority of them. However, there are some symptoms and signs that may prove difficult to recognize, so do not be surprised if, on some occasions, the iridologist refers to a text book.

During the 1940s, physical diagnosis reached its height. It was a time when the family doctor took an active part in your well-being. He referred you much less often to the impersonal hospital specialist. It was his task to produce a correct diagnosis and he would follow in the minutest detail every slight variation from the normal, just as a detective follows every clue in unravelling a mystery.

The iridologist has also been trained in the wealth of information that was documented and available from this time. This gives us further insight to the underlying bodily condition of the patient.

Iridologists and Their Work

Since the beginnings of iridology, those involved in research have endeavoured to link iris markings with specific organic diseases. As previously stated, it is not the intention of iris diagnosis to give a clinical diagnosis in the main. Yet it is often possible to identify specific iris signs that suggest certain bodily imbalances or disease processes which are occurring currently. It is then for the iridologist to identify the symptoms which accompany the particular illness and to take the appropriate action to help the patient towards better health.

It should be clear that it is not enough to see an iris marking without having the knowledge and understanding of its relevance to the body. It is indisputable that identifying only the marking would be a grave injustice to the patient. The student of iris-diagnosis is medically oriented, and requires the attributes of a teacher and friend as well as a doctor.

Modern iris researches have contributed immensely in the search for the truth; they have made available a wealth of information to iridologists who work in the field. Thus an experienced iridologist can, in turn, pass on these new benefits to their patients.

Ursula Sutter of Munich has studied the irises of children and from her work we now understand further the possible iris identification of:
1.   Certain bacteria in the body.
2.   Fermentive problems in children.
3.   Problems that occur with the lymphatic system in children.
4.   Response of the vegetative system.
5.   Calcifaction problems in children.

The iridologist Joachim Broy studied endocrinology and

became involved within the field of cybernetics. Cybernetics was first described by Norbert Wiener (1947), as 'a new name for a new science of the body's control and communication'. Broy's work has enhanced iris diagnosis in its early detection of hormonal problems.

Josef Angerer has probably contributed more to modern iridology than any other living iridologist. His work on the digestive system is unique and has listed many digestive hormones and their observation in the iris:

1. *Gastrin* is formed in the mucous membrane of the pylorus (opening from the stomach into the duodenum).
2. *Secretin* is a hormone secreted from the duodenum.
3. *Enterokinin* is formed in the mucous membrane of the small intestine and helps increase the enzymes in the jejunum and ileum. An iridological phenomenon occurs in what iridologists call a 'nasal frill'. This shows the loss of enzymes and with it a decrease of liquid matter and turbulences in the bowels.
4. *Parotin* is normally found in the sputum and in the parotid gland. However, it has now also been found in the membrane of the bowel. Absence of this hormone leads to impotence and its imbalance can be seen in the iris as a flattening of the pupil towards the nose.

Angerer also identified iris markings with liver hormones, one of which is heparin. This is an anticoagulant and is essential in keeping the blood flowing freely and preventing thrombosis. The marking for an absence of heparin is seen not in the iris, but in the sclera (the white of the eye). It is identified as brown coloured spots in a fatty, vein-filled mass which discolours the usual whiteness of the eye.

4

Iris Signs

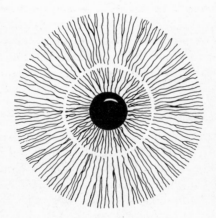

Figure 4.1   The iris

Lacunae, crypts, ladders, tulips and honeycombs are some of the colourful terms of iridology. Each variation of structure and each pattern shape seen in the iris has its own name for identification purposes. Not only is the structure important diagnostically but also the colour of the iris and pigmentations within the basic iris colour. These have their own meaning in relation to health and disease.

The eye is an extension of the brain yet it can be considered independent. From a hen's egg it is possible to detach the

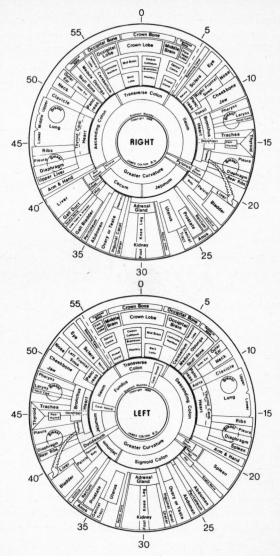

Figure 4.2   The British chart for clinical iris diagnosis

portion relating to the chick's eye and, by placing it in a jar and
giving it the correct growing medium, this little bud will grow
and develop into a complete chicken's eye with all its com-
plexities and light-sensitive chemicals. As bizarre as it sounds,
the eye is alive even though it is not connected to the chicken
or to its brain. The eye develops by genetic code from information carried by DNA (deoxyribonucleic acid) and the
messages of RNA (ribonucleic acid). Right at the beginning, at
conception, the iris is genetically programmed. This is the
very basis of iridology.

Circular Lacunae

Unlike the ordinary lacuna, this is rather less common and
when a circular lacuna appears in the pituitary gland zone of
the iris (as below), it indicates a disturbance of body fluids.
Patients may develop swollen feet and hands due to their body
retaining too much water. Such people usually look well-fed
but have a very pale skin.

Stress is always a major factor in these cases. Patients have a

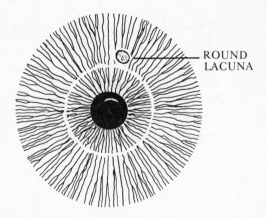

ROUND
LACUNA

Figure 4.3   Circular lacunae

low stress threshold and are more vulnerable to the pressures
of life.

Lacunae

The lacuna is a genetic marking and is termed a 'structural
marking'.

Lacunae are probably the most common of all iris markings. They are oval in shape and dislodge the surface layers of
the iris. They are either open or closed (see below) and are
found mainly in the kidney, pancreas and heart zones of
the iris.

Diagnostically they indicate organ insufficiency, clinically
they may never be seen to become evident. Ignaz von Peczely
said of them 'Hic signum – ubi ulcus?' (Here is the marking –
where is the problem?).

The German Iridologist Josef Deck called these signs
significant diagnosis of the iris lacuna. He found that problems often became clinically manifest after the organ was
damaged through infection or senility. If the kidney area is

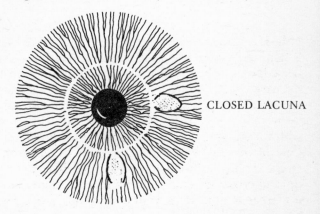

CLOSED LACUNA

OPEN LACUNA

Figure 4.4   Closed and open lacunae

damaged by a blow to the lower back, it is more likely that the patient will develop kidney problems if there is a lacuna present in the corresponding zone of the iris.

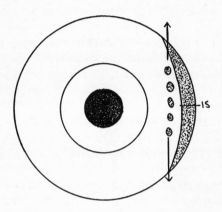

Figure 4.5 Pale flecks

Pale Flecks

When pale flecks such as these appear in front of a darkened iris edge, it indicates a problem in the function of the skin.

Years ago, iridologists believed these pale flecks showed lymphatic disturbances but we now know that they indicate poor skin reaction. There may also be problems associated with the lungs and bronchia such as emphysema or asthma. One of my patients who showed this type of iris marking, suffered with both her lungs and her skin. Every winter she developed dry eczema and whenever she had a cold, if she did not treat it quickly, it would develop into a nasty bout of pleurisy. By taking a mixture of pleurisy root, ginger, comfrey and licorice, she was subsequently able to avoid anything serious from developing.

Daisy Iris

This is one of the most distinctive iris markings and gets its
name from the close resemblance in shape to the flower.
Although any iris sign may be seen in both blue and brown
eyes, this one is frequently observed in those with blue eyes. It
is a quite commonly seen sign and indicates genetic disposition to general glandular disturbances. Quite often there
is a family history of diabetes, and the iridologist will always
investigate this aspect.

We find that if there are no physical signs of diabetes, and
blood tests prove negative, the patient nearly always experiences
a particular series of symptoms; headaches, dizzy spells, shaking
and trembling, extreme hunger, sugar cravings, sweating and
palpitations. The medical term for these symptoms of low
blood sugar is hypoglycaemia. This can be treated successfully
by a dietary approach and supplements to suit the individual.

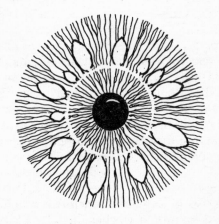

Figure 4.6   Daisy iris

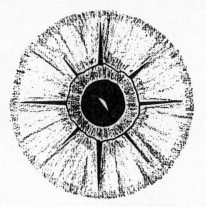

Figure 4.7   Asthenic ridges

Asthenic Ridges
Asthenic ridges are identified as black lines radiating around
the iris. This is one of the few iris markings which can change
visibly. The ridges indicate low energy and poor nerve supply
to the organ in which corresponding iris zone they appear. If,
for example, an asthenic ridge appeared in the adrenal zone of
your iris you would undoubtedly be feeling extra tired, lacking
energy and vitality, sometimes with a lack of appetite.
Occasionally, depression and irritability is a feature. Salt craving
may accompany these symptoms and would be taken into
account by the iridologist before treatment was advised. Many
of our patients benefit from acupuncture treatment to re-
establish the energy flow to the whole body.

The Tulip Sign
This sign consists of a thick fibre which splits into a definite
tulip shape by the time it reaches the edge of the iris. When
such a sign appears in the upper part of the iris, usually in the
sinus zones, it indicates intercranial problems. Most often this

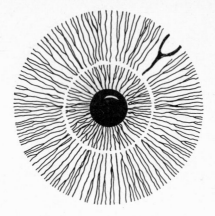

Figure 4.8   The tulip sign

sign is accompanied by frontal headache, loss of smell and occasionally dizziness. These are frequent symptoms of sinusitis and, if left untreated, could lead to more serious disease such as otitis media (inflammation of the middle ear), acute bronchitis, asthma, meningitis and pneumonia. Treatment for sinusitis, especially in its early stages, can be accomplished by applying infra-red heat over the sinus area. The aim is to drain the nasal cavity and, in some congenital abnormalities, drainage is possible only when the person is upside down. Excluding this condition, even the most stubborn case will respond to Poke Root (Phytolocca Decandra).

Transversal

This is a single fibre that runs astray, not by accident but by design. More commonly seen in the lower half of the iris, it indicates a change to the particular organ or structure through which it runs. One such organ zone where we often see this marking is the liver. It is then of vital importance that every aspect of the patient's health is discovered.

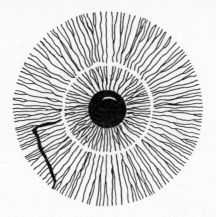

Figure 4.9   A transversal

Occasionally, a transversal is observed in the spinal zone of the iris when there is a curvature, either to the left or right, of the spine. Such cases would need the treatment of an osteopath or chiropractor.

The Honeycomb
Honeycomb signs appear exactly as the name suggests, small hexagonal clusters. Although they can be seen anywhere in the iris structure, the most frequent zones are lungs, uterus, kidneys and bladder.

It is a sign which is determined genetically and indicates degeneration of the organ. If the honeycomb is seen in the lung zone, the iridologist will ascertain the extent of any lung or breathing disorder. Wheezing, persistent coughs or difficult breathing are the sort of symptoms associated with the honeycomb. People who have a family incidence of tuberculosis frequently show this sign.

As a general rule, the corresponding organ of the body which shows the honeycomb will be included in any treatment,

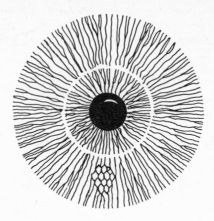

Figure 4.10   The honeycomb

even if there are no physical symptoms manifesting at the time. If it is the lung in question, herbs such as coltsfoot, horehound and pleurisy root will be given.

The drawings on the preceding pages are just a few of the many markings and signs seen in the iris. There are about two hundred different signs in all and they include variations of colour and pigment spots.

Identifying iris signs accurately takes many years of practice and the correlation between the sign and the bodily condition requires a broad understanding of how the body works. It is not enough for the practitioner simply to name the sign. He must be able to explain the underlying cause of what is going wrong in the body before he can correct it with treatment. Because it is possible to pin-point past disease and old injuries, the psychological effect on the patient is spectacular and creates a unique relationship between the patient and the practitioner.

Often some of our patients cannot remember all their past

health problems during the consultation. It is only later, when they have spoken to relatives that they remember the broken arm or the rheumatic fever they had as a child.

5

What the Iris Cannot Reveal

There have been some attempts to disprove the validity of iris diagnosis. One such attempt was made in 1956 by two German doctors, Kibler and Sterzing, who claimed to be researching iris diagnosis. They published an article stating that there was nothing in iris diagnosis, even though they did not have even a basic knowledge of iridology. Many of their own colleagues, including Professor Schnell, asked them repeatedly to work with an iridologist which they refused to do. Their main objection to iridology's validity was that childhood infections such as measles, chicken pox and mumps did not show in the iris. However, iridologists had known for hundreds of years that the iris does not show infections. If Kibler and Sterzing had taken their colleagues' advice and worked with an iridologist, they could have saved themselves the time and trouble of researching something that we already knew!

However, the problems facing iridology are not from scientific research (we welcome this) but from those who claim to be able to see some magical and mystical signs from the eyes. The eyes have always been associated, to some extent, with the soul. Indeed, when we are introduced to someone, we instinctively focus on their eyes to try to assess their character. We feel uneasy when someone will not look at us when they are talking to us. Receded and indented eyelids usually mean the person has a quick temper. Strongly bulging eyes are commonly found on highly talkative people. However, it is the expression of the eyes which is considered the most important physionomical sign. A sweet look bears witness to a soft personality, a fleeting and lively look indicates a sensitive and apprehensive soul. It is obvious that we can all, to some extent, judge a person's character by the shape of the whole eye apparatus. It can be great fun to try to determine a partner's or friend's personality in this way. The iris *does not* by any stretch of the imagination display the inner soul, the personality, or whether you will meet a tall, dark stranger! On the other hand, every iridologist will know the physiological effects some organs have on the brain, so influencing the mind and personality. The liver is one such organ and in one particular liver disease, the personality changes because toxic material interferes with the brain's functions causing mental dullness and confusion. The pancreas is another organ which can bring about a change in personality. In hypoglycaemia (low blood sugar), the brain receives reduced supplies of vital glucose. Patients change from being calm and orderly to having periods of extreme tension, panic attacks and disordered thought patterns.

Deficiencies of vital nutrients also have an undesirable effect on personality and mood. An irritable baby who cries when he or she is handled and who is a difficult feeder may have a vitamin C deficiency. When the vitamin is introduced the baby will become calm and relaxed. Inadequate daily amounts of the B group of vitamins may result in poor sleep patterns and a slow learning ability. Hormones, food allergies and many other factors play their part in determining mood and personality.

Identification of some personality problems lies in the ability to understand the physiological effects on the brain.

A mother brought her fourteen year old son to see us because he was aggressive, irritable, deceptive and had general behavioural problems. We put a total ban on sugar and products containing sugar. He visited us twice-weekly to strengthen his resolve and, within six weeks, he was a changed person. Gone was any trace of aggression, he helped around the house, had taken up a school sport and even his teacher had a good word for him!

On another occasion a thirty-year-old man, who was under the complete dominance of his widowed mother, sought our help for digestive problems. The cause was obvious and, after counselling him and his mother, he went hiking in Scotland for two months which was his great passion. His mother moved into a smaller bungalow, something she had always wanted to do. When we opened the door to him some ten weeks later, we did not recognize him. He stood tall when he had slouched, had lost weight, his digestive problems had disappeared, an obviously changed man.

Hic Signum Ubi Ulcus? (Here is the Marking, Where is the Problem?)

Von Peczely knew that what he had stumbled on by accident was a truly fantastic diagnostic aid. He knew that, for the first time, the patient could be seen in his total wholeness – past, present and future.

This problem of seeing the marking in the iris but without any significant clinical findings, caused von Peczely to spend the better part of his life researching the iris. He was already at a grave disadvantage for his equipment consisted solely of a 2 x magnifying glass. However, given the benefits of today's sophisticated cameras and biomicroscopes, his research might have been quite different. Like Leonardo da Vinci, Peczely was born way ahead of his time. None the less, there remained one question that he could not answer. He found that when a patient had a particular iris marking in the gastrointestinal zone which indicated an ulcer, it did not necessarily mean the patient had a gastrointestinal ulcer at that time. This is a phenomenon which faces iridologists daily and this is why it is sometimes necessary to monitor a patient for many years. It may be important to have an iris picture taken for examination each year.

Von Peczely never came to terms with this problem and became disillusioned. He knew many years of dedicated research were still needed before this would be explained. He became vulnerable to criticism and was depressed in later life. When his end finally came he instructed his family 'spread my ashes and extinguish my name!'. This was a sad ending for one so dedicated in helping the sick and dying. However, others took up the challenge and performed their own research. One such pioneer was German-born Josef Deck. In 1935 he faced this situation on his own and was to spend the better part of his life researching this problem. In the 1950s he called a meeting of the experts in ocular research to unite iridologists in the search for the answer to 'Hic signum ubi ulcus?' Problems occurred in financing this research; private research is always costly and no money was available either from business or the state.

Unable to resolve these money matters with his medical colleagues, Deck found himself alone again. Then fate stepped in and provided him with the answer.

One of Deck's friends, a well-known professor of medicine asked him to examine his iris. Deck found the iris marking in question in the left upper abdominal zone. The professor was not experiencing symptoms connected with what the iris showed. Eleven years later an unexpected perforation occurred and partial gastrectomy was necessary. Deck had found the answer. These markings were *latent* markings. He monitored other patients with this type of iris marking and they all developed similar symptoms at a later stage in their life.

People go periodically to the dentist to have their teeth examined for decay. It is also important that they should occasionally visit an iridologist to have their iris examined to check that vital organs are working harmoniously. If the dentist discovers a cavity it is hardly life-threatening but, if minor bodily imbalances can be corrected, a serious disease may be avoided. An ounce of prevention is worth a pound of cure.

All too often the iridologist is asked to clarify a condition that has already manifested itself into a serious illness. We were once asked to diagnose a sergeant in the army. In typical army style he gave us only his name, rank and number and refused to discuss his health until the consultation was over. Only slightly deterred, we conducted the diagnosis and took his iris photograph in the normal way. Our diagnosis was: serious problem in the liver, heart and pancreas with irritation markings in the urinary zones. He confirmed his – he had a serious disease called haemochromatosis (Bronzed Diabetes). This is a hereditary disorder in which there is excessive absorption and storage of iron. It affects the liver, pancreas and, eventually, the heart finally causing death. The irritation to the urinary tract which we had discovered turned out to be a recent prostrate and renal pelvic problem. He was not looking for a miracle cure or even treatment and why he came we were not sure – perhaps he just wanted the diagnosis confirmed.

Pregnancy

We have sometimes been asked if pregnancy can be detected from the iris. The simple answer is, no. However, it is often possible to see problems that may cause difficulties during the pregnancy. Already weak kidneys will need extra care at this time to help avoid toxaemia of pregnancy or high blood pressure. If the iris shows a tendency towards poor circulation, advice may be given to help prevent varicose veins from forming in the legs. However, the actual pregnancy will not be recorded in the iris. Any naturally-occurring phenomena will not show in the iris.

This can also be true of accidents where bones have been

broken. Patients sometimes show concern when a past skiing accident is not seen by the iridologist. Often the patient's in-built constitution has dealt quite adequately with the trauma and stress of the injury, leaving no sign in the iris, or at least a marking the iridologist feels has no significance.

Because iris diagnosis may appear to be simplistic it has made an impression on the minds of many, from those dedicated to the promotion of wellness, to those merely curious of a new approach.

Our passion and belief in the truth push us on. We will not give up the quest to make iridology available, freely, to all those who require the benefits that this system of diagnosis has to offer.

6

The Right Road to Health

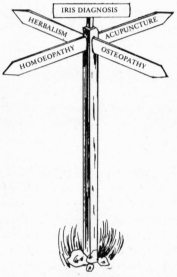

Figure 6.1   The right road to health

Each branch of the healing arts offers its own method of treatment. Osteopathy centres its treatment on manipulation of the skeletal structure of the body, and can treat many conditions including those of the gallbladder, kidneys and stomach via manipulation. A herbalist would treat the same conditions of the gallbladder, kidneys and stomach along with other conditions but, instead of using manipulative treatments, he would administer specific herbs to strengthen the body's own healing powers.

A homoeopath treats illness by administering extremely small doses of substances that in large doses would bring about similar symptoms to the original illness. The onion is well known for causing runny noses and eyes but, in minute doses, the onion is a good cold remedy when similar symptoms appear.

An acupuncturist will treat illnesses by correcting the energy flow to vital organs via the meridians and, together with homoeopathy, is one of the few alternative therapies to be found in the British National Health system.

Allopathic medicine treats illness by administering chemicals that have been scientifically proved and are known to bring about various alterations in the body's functions. Although many of these drugs are life-saving in certain emergencies, they all have undesirable side-effects. Often surgery is used to remove diseased organs that allopathic medicine cannot treat.

When considering all these excellent therapies, how do you decide which system of treatment would be most beneficial? Usually patients seek alternative treatment when they find no help from their family doctor and the numbers are growing daily. Most patients consult an alternative practitioner because of a recommendation from a friend who has received successful treatment. However, such faith does not necessarily mean the treatment offered is the best system suited to your needs.

Iridology knows. Iris diagnosis will point you in the right direction, individually suited to your needs. Iridologists have the ability and experience to treat a wide range of illness but they may decide the spinal problem found in the iris should be treated by an osteopath, the liver dysfunction by a herbalist. Referrals may range from an osteopath to a reflexologist, from a herbalist to a doctor, or from a homoeopath to yoga therapy.

A lady once consulted us for a long-term health problem. She initially wrote to me asking for a consultation: 'I have suffered severe tiredness (with accompanying problems) for at least the last twelve years. I have sought the help of orthodox medicine over the past five years and I am not over-stating it when I say that I am the most diagnosed person in the UK but without any results. I have been diagnosed as having a hormonal imbalance, suffering from hypoglycaemia, food allergies (such as being diagnosed as a coeliac), allergy to dairy products and, lastly, allergy to animal fat. All these diagnoses have subsequently been proved incorrect but, unfortunately, whilst all this is going on I am reduced to a mere existence (for twelve years). I have sought and fought hard to help myself and I am almost certain that my problem is not food allergies . . .'

Her iris showed a hormone imbalance, a genetic heart problem (this was later confirmed by her doctor) and a spinal problem which we considered to be the reason for her symptoms. We prescribed the herb Agnus Castus (Vitex Agnus-Castus) to help correct the hormone imbalance and suggested manipulation therapy. We recommended her to the clinic run in London by the British School of Osteopathy and are pleased to say that after just a few visits, she began to regain her health and strength.

On the other hand, the iridologist may already be a practising osteopath and therefore he will be in a position to treat the spinal problem himself, referring you to a herbalist for correcting the hormone imbalance. Usually the iridologist is experienced in one or more branches of the healing arts so would be able to treat you himself but he will always know when to refer.

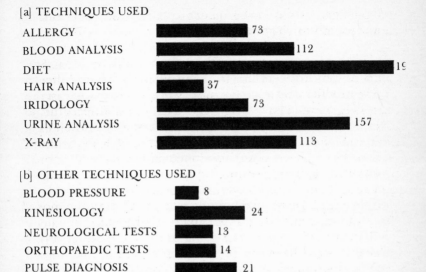

[a] TECHNIQUES USED

ALLERGY	73
BLOOD ANALYSIS	112
DIET	19
HAIR ANALYSIS	37
IRIDOLOGY	73
URINE ANALYSIS	157
X-RAY	113

[b] OTHER TECHNIQUES USED

BLOOD PRESSURE	8
KINESIOLOGY	24
NEUROLOGICAL TESTS	13
ORTHOPAEDIC TESTS	14
PULSE DIAGNOSIS	21
RADIONICS	7
TONGUE DIAGNOSIS	17

Diagnostic techniques used

Practitioners were asked to indicate, from a choice of seven different techniques, any that they used in reaching a diagnosis (Figure 12). X-ray was used mainly by chiropractors (94), although some osteopaths (10) and naturopaths (4) also use this technique. A little under half (193) of the respondents (411) use dietary analysis, particularly naturopaths (80% of those practising naturopathy as their main therapy) and herbalists (64%). Of the practitioners who use blood tests, herbalists (42%) and chiropractors (40%) tended to use these more than other practitioners. Herbalists (79%) also use urine tests most frequently, followed by naturopaths (53%) and chiropractors (48%). Hair analysis was the least used technique, being used by only 9% of the total sample. Allergy testing was used predominantly by naturopaths (47%) and herbalists (45%). Iridology was employed most by homoeopaths (50%).

Figure 6.2 Diagram illustrating the numbers of practitioners using (a) one or more of the seven named techniques to help reach a diagnosis; (b) other techniques

The Institute for Complementary Medicine recently brought out a report called *Trends in Complementary Medicine*. The report consists of various data collected from 411 practitioners from the major branches of complementary medicine. It showed that 73 practitioners use iridology as a diagnostic tool. Of these fifty per cent were homoeopaths, and the numbers are growing. It could be that the majority of practitioners of all the disciplines, although not registered, are using iridology to enhance their diagnostic skills. However, amongst the different branches of alternative medicine, it is undoubtedly homoeopaths who understand the principles and find the greatest benefit of iridology as a diagnostic tool. This is not surprising as continental homoeopaths have used iridology as their main diagnostic tool for many, many years.

The importance of diagnosing an illness pattern *before* it becomes a major health problem is obvious; it can save not only untold misery and pain but life itself. We have all seen a young man or woman who has abused their body with alcohol, drugs (both prescribed and non-prescribed), poor nutrition or an unhealthy life-style and maybe their attitude to 'health' is non-existent, saying 'Why bother taking vitamins; I might be run over by a bus tomorrow'.

This kind of irresponsible reasoning leaves us cold for it is this very type of person who is programming himself for serious illness at a later stage in his life. One such debilitating illness is dementia of which there are two types. One is senile dementia in which the functioning part of the brain becomes degenerative causing the loss of intellectual facilities. In some cases senile dementia can be detected genetically. The other form of dementia is arteriosclerotic. This causes the brain to degenerate because the blood supply becomes impaired. Arteriosclerotic dementia is a pitiful condition – happy one moment, crying the next and falling into deep pits of depression. Antidepressants are usually prescribed or electrotherapy applied. Patients commonly fall prey to strokes and hypertension, and the incidence of epilepsy is higher than average. Not a satisfactory condition and certainly not one that we would wish upon ourselves or others. However, considering that a staggering ten per cent of all old people suffer from dementia, half of them severely (and in the over-eighties the proportion rises to one in five) it seems that many of us will fall victim to this disease. Yet, in nearly all cases, if caught in time this terrible condition could be prevented. It must put *prevention* and very early *detection* at the top of the list.

Doctors are well aware of the social problems this condition brings with it, for there are few conditions that tax both the family and the doctor as these sad cases do. Patience and understanding is often lacking, frustration takes over and creates friction between patient, relatives and the doctor. However, some doctors have been trying to find ways to help. Research with lecithin has brought to light phosphatidyl choline – an active component of lecithin. This has been shown to be useful in the treatment of arteriosclerosis. In 1978 Dr F. Etienne in Montreal studied seven patients with Alzheimer's disease, a progressive form of dementia, sometimes called presenile dementia because it usually begins in middle age. Dr Etienne and some of his colleagues artifically increased the amount of choline in patients' blood by giving lecithin. They then tested the effect and efficiency of their learning ability. The results were remarkable; three out of the original seven showed an increased learning ability, noticeably clearer speech and all scored higher points on a learning test. It seems clear that lecithin can help in personality.

People who are found to be susceptible to this form of dementia can prevent it manifesting into a major health problem. Simply cutting out saturated fats (hard fats) salt and stopping smoking and instead, introducing foods high in lecithin, such as soy bean oil, can mean a happy and active retirement.

Smoking is probably one of the easiest ways to get lung

cancer; it also hits the top in the prevention charts. Stop smoking and you extend your life by years and probably contribute to saving resources that could be put to better medical use. Think how important iris diagnosis would be to those smokers who persist with the habit to be told of a genetic flaw in their lungs which would increase their chance of developing lung cancer.

7

Other Eye Problems

The iridologist is not an ophthalmologist. However, it is of vital importance that the iris diagnostician can recognize simple eye diseases and be familiar with their treatment. When an eye disorder or disease is suspected, the patient is usually referred to an ophthalmologist for further examination. Sometimes, treating a simple eye disorder can be easy and a matter of common sense.

I remember an elderly lady who came to see me some years ago, for iris diagnosis. She was not feeling unwell but she was keen that she should retain her good health. I remember her well as she was a joy to meet and she evidently enjoyed life to the full. I could find little wrong with her. She had very few genetic weaknesses, had never had surgery of any kind and had always kept to a good, simple diet with plenty of fresh food. Apart from accidents, there was absolutely no reason why she should not continue her good health for some time to come. There was just one problem. Headaches. I spent about twenty minutes investigating the root cause but came up with a blank. I had been looking at this lady for about an hour now, but it was only when she took her spectacles off and absently rubbed her eyes did I suspect what the trouble could be. Her newly fitted spectacles were not correct. The next day she returned to her optician, her spectacles were changed and her headaches disappeared.

Simple eye problems like this can often be rectified with the help of an iridologist who will be familiar with the way the eye works. He often can see the very early stages of more serious disorders such as cataracts, glaucoma, pterygium and other diseases.

Glaucoma

It is particularly important to detect the early stages of chronic glaucoma where the pressure inside the eyeball is raised. Normally the patient is quite unaware that anything is wrong until there is actual damage to the eye and vision begins to fail. In the early stages there is normally no change in visual ability, no pain or discomfort, but the iridologist may be able to detect a slight colour change to the pupil. This is especially easy to observe when examining a second or subsequent iris photograph which has been taken at a later date and, by comparing with the original, early changes are spotted at once. Symptoms of simple glaucoma are often absent but, by the time the disease has progressed, patients report seeing haloes around electric lights, and vision which is worse during the evening and at night. By now pain is present in the eye and headaches are common. In severe cases vomiting may lead the patient to suspect a digestive upset.

One of the ways to help with early detection of glaucoma is always to make sure your optician checks your eyes for this disease. It is a very simple test and one which you should ask for when having your normal yearly check-up. We always advise our patients to have it; glaucoma can damage your sight irrevocably, so it is well worth taking positive steps for its early detection. The test involves a small puff of air being blown onto the eye and a machine registers the response time of your blink. Drops may then be prescribed to help reduce the pressure in the eye. Herbal remedies may also be helpful.

This is a story related to us by a patient who had had acute glaucoma and found herself with night blindness. She woke one night to visit the bathroom and could see nothing at all. She switched on her bedside light and, when it did not come on, she thought the bulb had broken. Switching on the landing light, which also did not come on, she thought a fuse had caused the lights to fail. Untroubled she returned to bed. In the morning she realized the lights were perfectly all right. Unfortunately she did not realize the significance of her night blindness which continued for several weeks. It was only on a chance visit to her optician, who happened to work at Moorfield's Eye Hospital, that glaucoma was found and subsequently treated.

Cataracts

There are several causes of cataracts and they can also follow many diseases. Old age is said to be one cause (although we believe it more likely to be due to nutritional deficiencies). If the metabolism goes wrong or if trauma to the eye occurs, cataracts can develop.

A lady once visited us for a consultation. She had been repairing an old chair and was removing the tacks with a screwdriver when one of them flicked up and pierced her eye. She had no choice but to pull it out herself. Straightaway she went to an eye hospital to receive help and treatment, but the damage was already done and a traumatic cataract had formed. We wanted to say to her that she had been careless and should have worn safety goggles but I suppose we all take chances at times – only this time fate was against her.

Detection of a cataract can sometimes be revealed in an iris photograph but the best way to see opaqueness of the lens in the eye is by using a ophthalmoscope. This allows the operator to see the early cataract as a grey or black shadow against the 'red pupillary reflex'.

Unfortunately the allopathic system has no way of treating an early cataract. You have to wait until the cataract is advanced, until the crystalline lens is no longer clear but opaque like a pearl. Then the cataract is termed 'ripe' and the lens is removed surgically.

We have seen the results of some amazing surgical techniques where an artificial lens has been fitted into the eye. However, this may be traumatic for the patient especially as there may be blindness in one eye, yet having to wait months for an operation. On the other hand, it is very rewarding to treat early cataracts with herbal and nutritional remedies. Research by Allen Taylor of Tufts University Laboratory for Nutrition and Cataract Department in Massachusetts, revealed that the eye contains a staggering 30 times more vitamin C than the blood. He also found that by substantially raising vitamin C levels, cataracts would become retarded in their progression to blindness.

Cancer

A study on 2,000 Americans found that certain people were more likely to develop cancer of the eye than others. Babies and young children who were exposed to strong sunlight have a greater chance of developing eye cancer in later life. Those with blue eyes are 60% more at risk than those with brown eyes.

The problem seems to stem from short exposure to intense sunlight rather than longer exposure to moderate sunlight. If you are visiting warmer, sunnier climates either for a holiday, or on business, and you have blue eyes, wear a good pair of polarized sun-glasses. Do not risk the health of your eyes by wearing cheap tinted glasses; they may actually do more harm than good by causing the pupil to dilate letting in *more*, not less, sunlight. Whether young children have blue eyes or not, they should be protected with a hat or bonnet which shades their face.

Pterygium

Although a pterygium is usually harmless to normal vision they do worry patients mainly because they are unsightly. They start in the conjunctiva (white of the eye) and, for a reason we do not yet fully understand, nearly always occur on the nasal side of the eye. As a small mass of fibrous blood vessels it grows, pushing a gelatinous tip towards the pupil, over the cornea, until it invades the pupil and affects the vision. Its cause is unknown although some specialists link its cause with actinic light (short-wave radiant energy that causes chemical changes). Others have found that pterygium occurs more frequently in windy, dusty climates. Surgical removal has so far been the only treatment available.

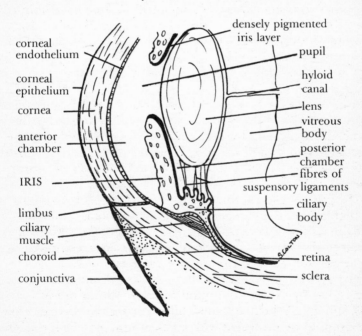

Figure 7.1   Structure of the eye

Please note:
If you think you have something wrong with the function of
your eyes, or a disorder or disease, consult an ophthalmologist
without delay.

8

Constitutional Types

Constitutional factors affect just about every aspect of our make-up (our character, physical shape, hair colour and pre-sition to certain diseases). People have been grouped er by types which have been categorized in various ways.

In Chinese medicine, Yang and Yin are the positive and negative aspects of constitution. As heat is to cold, Yang is to Yin. Yang is masculine, Yin is feminine. In order for perfect health to be achieved, a correct balance between Yang and Yin must be obtained. In homoeopathic medicine, patients are grouped according to their symptoms and the remedy which is indicated. Homoeopaths throughout the world refer to their patients as being a 'sulphur case' or a 'Pulsatilla case' and so on. This is because the patient's set of symptoms indicate the name of the remedy to be used most effectively. The 'sulphur' patient is lean, lank and hungry, suffers indigestion and has stooped shoulders. If the patient is a child, his face will look dirty even though it has just been washed. The sulphur scholar works day and night, not caring for order or food.

Categories

Until quite recently (about 1940) the allopathic system of medicine used external characteristic signs in diagnosing disease, and patients were categorized into different bodily configurations as follows:

Sthenic Type
This type is characterized by a short, stocky frame, broad chest and a short neck. The hands are broad with short, stumpy fingers and the person is considered to have good physical strength.

Asthenic Type
These types are tall, have a long neck with a long flat chest, and a protruding abdomen. The hands are slender and the fingers long. A sub group of this category is the so-called neurasthenic the neurotic type who complain of a tight band around the head, have sexual problems and are subject to abdominal problems. They are easily tired, mentally and physically.

Plethoric Type
The plethoric type are of short stature, have a broad chest with a rather short neck similar to the first type. However, the plethoric type have a disproportionately large waistline. Their complexion is flushed or ruddy and they always seem to have suffused and watery eyes. They are prone to renal, cardio-vascular and respiratory problems.

Phthisical Type
This type are said to be an exaggerated form of the asthenic category and often have chest deformities with the bones of the chest standing out. Nutrition is often poor and wasting may occur.

We all fall into constitutional types and can be 'fitted' into one category or another.

Fingerprints
Fingerprints have long been associated with crime because of their uniqueness but they also have a place in medicine. There are six distinctive pattern formations to be found on the fingertips:

1. Double loops.
2. Tented loop.
3. Radial loop.
4. Arch.
5. Whorl.
6. Ulnar loop.

Patterns on the fingers, palms of the hand, the toes and soles of the feet, are all unique to each of us. Dermatoglyphics is the name for this science. It is of great value not only to doctors but also anthropologists studying genetics. Like your iris, your fingerprints could show you to which constitutional type you belong.

Considering fingerprints can show many inherited diseases, it is hardly surprising that the sensitive eye shows so much more. After all, fingerprints are relatively simple in their pattern formation and have little colour variation. The iris far exceeds this simplicity. With highly complex structural patterns and a great many colour variations, the iris is available for examination. It gives iridology strong grounds for further investigation even by those with 'closed minds'. If a diagnosis can be obtained without intervention by drugs, surgery or X-ray, it must, surely, be worthy of further study.

By the same criteria for fingerprints, the iris has also provided accurate and complex information about an individual constitution.

Each constitutional type has its own iris colour, iris structure symptoms and disposition to certain diseases. The iridologist will be familiar with all these groups and subgroups; they give him an immediate insight to your family's medical history. If your iris showed a urinary diathesis, it is more likely that one or both your parents had some kind of arthritis, rheumatism or gout. Of course this does not mean that you will inevitably suffer with arthritis but it does mean that you will have a tendency to do so.

THE MAIN CONSTITUTIONAL TYPES

Lymphatic, Haematogenous and Biliary

These are then subdivided into ten smaller groups:

MAIN GROUP		THEIR SUBGROUPS
Lymphatic	1.	Pure Lymphatic.
	2.	Hydrogenoid.
	3.	Urinary diathesis.
	4.	Lipaemic diathesis.
	5.	Neurogenic.
Haematogenous	1.	Pure Haematogenous.
	2.	Lavate tetanic.
Biliary (mixed)	1.	Biliary (mixed).
	2.	Ferrum-chromatosis.
	3.	Weak connective tissue.

If your iris colour is a deep, rich brown (which is characteristic of the haematogenous constitutional type) you are less likely to suffer the pains and discomfort of arthritis but instead, constitutionally, you will have a tendency towards blood disorders which may involve the heart and kidneys and you may find you lack sufficient iron and copper.

PREDISPOSITION TO DISEASE

TYPE	IRIS STRUCTURE	LIKELY DISEASE
Lymphatic	The colour is usually light blue and may appear to be a darker shade at the outer edge of the iris. There is a distinctly light ring around the frill. The iris fibres are	There is usually a susceptibility to catarrh and disease of the lymphatic system and infections of the upper respiratory tract. In children, tonsils, adenoids

arranged at random, some appearing tightly stretched. and lungs are vulnerable.

Haematogenous The colour is deep, rich brown and is sometimes called 'the velvet carpet'. Under magnification, only a few iris features are seen.

Diseases are often of the glandular system and of the blood which may involve the heart and kidneys due to the characteristic lack of trace elements such as iron and copper.

Biliary (mixed) The colour usually appears as mid-brown and is often mistaken for 'hazel' eyes. When magnified, the deeper iris layers appear blue. There are often quite large patches of blue showing through. A person with this eye colour will often claim that their eyes change colour.

As the name suggests, diseases of the biliary tract and liver are indicated.

It is often possible to determine the future health trends of a young child especially when the parents' and sometimes the grandparents' iris constitutions have been determined.

9

Case Histories

The following case histories were taken from our clinic files. Any branch of medicine will demonstrate their patients who have overcome illnesses with the aid of that particular branch of medicine. However, with the possible exception of surgery, the majority of patients seeking the specific help of an iridologist have tried other forms of healing with little or no improvement.

Case History 1
William, aged 59 and a retired engineer, was of average height and weighed 65 kg (140 lb). Some years ago he had had a perforated ulcer. Although surgery had saved his life, the operation had unfortunately removed two thirds of his digestive tract. Consequently, William was having digestive problems. He was also developing arthritis in his hands; small hard nodules could be seen under his skin. Having spent a great deal of time and energy trying to find relief he came, as a last desperate attempt, to find help.

His iris showed depletion of bacteria that help in the digestive processes. His body was very low in zinc and for this reason we prescribed 60 mg of zinc to be taken daily for one month. *Lacto bacillus acidophilus* was recommended as a long-term digestive aid, together with specific herbs chaparral and prickly ash bark. We also advised daily dosages of vitamin C 2g, pantothenic acid 200 mg vitamin A 10,000 iu's and

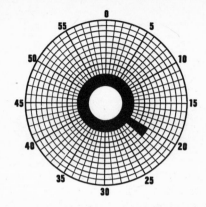

Figure 9.1   Case history 1: William's iris

vitamin D 400 iu's. The dietary advice we offered included a drastic reduction of alcohol, tea and coffee, and the introduction of more fresh fruit and vegetables. After two months William returned and told us that his digestive problems had improved dramatically and that the nodules on his hands had begun to disappear.

Case History 2
Carrie, a 13 year old schoolgirl, came for iris diagnosis to see whether the cause of a long-standing headache could be revealed. Three years previously she had fallen backwards onto the edge of an old fashioned iron bedstead, hitting the back of her head. Despite many investigations, X-rays and drug therapy, Carrie always had a headache. She could not take part in school sports activity as she found the headache became much worse. At times, all she could do was lie down for a few days until the pain eased a little.

Her iris showed irritation and inflammation in the left skull and cervical zones. We suspected structural lesions in both these areas. After taking chiropractic and massage treatment,

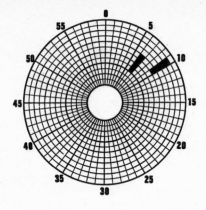

Figure 9.2   Case history 2: Carrie's iris

the pain reduced by more than half. She was able to take part in her school sports once again and concentrate on her lessons. Vitamin E and B complex were prescribed and treatment continues in order to reduce the pain level further.

Case History 3
Zac is a 30 year old computer technical analyst. He came to see us because of problems he was having with both mental and physical symptoms. These included extreme tiredness, intestinal gas, abdominal bloating and discomfort with periods of diarrhoea and constipation. Eating certain foods seemed to upset him and he had sugar, bread and beer cravings. He also suspected food allergies. His muscles ached and were stiff during normal activity. He felt anxious, depressed, irritable, had difficulty in thinking clearly, and in concentrating even over short periods. Finally, he had experienced memory loss. This might sound an amazing list of symptoms but Zac's iris revealed but one cause.

When an organ is not functioning correctly, there is usually a particular set of symptoms. Some may be subtle and not

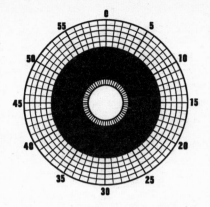

Figure 9.3   Case history 3: Zac's iris

generally related to another. Zac's iris showed the classic sign for Candida Overgrowth Syndrome.

His condition was improved by avoiding yeast, foods containing yeast products, foods made by fermentation (such as beer), and taking a variety of vitamins and minerals, including vitamin C, zinc, garlic and acidophilus.

Case History 4
Ted, a 42 year old fitter, came to see us because his wife had been diagnosed a few weeks previously. He was having difficulty in sleeping. However, the main problem, which he had suffered for 15 years, was that he always felt tired even when he was not working. He had dull pain in the lower back, and extremely 'restless legs'; he could not sit for more than an hour without having to walk about.

Ted's iris showed three problems. The first was a kidney malfunction (the dull pain in the lower back). Secondly, there was a cholesterol ring and, when seen with the third problem, an iris marking in the liver zone showed a serious disturbance in the fat metabolism. In Ted's case this was producing high

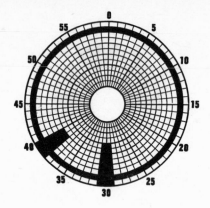

Figure 9.4   Case history 4: Ted's iris

blood cholesterol and giving him his 'restless legs'. However, by knowing the root cause of his symptoms, treatment was much more effective. He quickly improved with a course of vitamins and minerals to suit his individual needs.

Case History 5
Walter, a 49 year old self-employed builder, was successful and proud of it. He was tall, slim and of a nervous disposition, claiming that smoking calmed him down. He was going through a family crisis which he found difficult to handle. He had stomach pain (the burning type) and often felt he had cramp in his stomach. Sometimes his sleep was disturbed around 2.00 am. He was always careful about the food he ate but could not find out the cause of his suspected allergy.

Quite often patients come to see us because they suspect a food allergy. Sometimes this is disproved by iris diagnosis. In Walter's case we immediately saw the iris sign which was confirming his distress. A crypt (a small black mark) was clearly visible in the duodenal zone and indicated a duodenal ulcer.

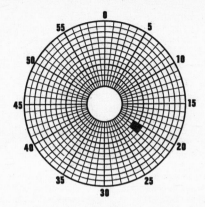

Figure 9.5   Case history 5: Walter's iris

By giving him a combination of comfrey, marshmallow root, golden seal powder, poke root and cransbill herbs, all his stomach symptoms disappeared.

Case History 6

Nora was 52 when she came for iris diagnosis. She had suffered with severe, chronic diarrhoea for several months. This had now resulted in her feeling very weak and debilitated. Her iris revealed that her colon was extremely inflamed and producing mucous which is normally associated with mucous colitis. Further talks with Nora revealed that she was undergoing a separation from her husband. She did not want the separation and was desperately trying to patch up the relationship. Her stress levels were very high. Again, this is quite common in cases of mucous colitis. Her iris also showed a congenital heart defect; she had had a heart problem when she was nine years old.

Nora's symptoms disappeared when we gave her zinc, along with other vitamins and minerals. We also introduced a little natural oil into her diet, which was to consist mainly of

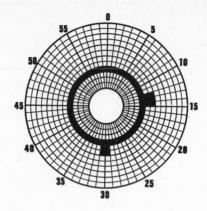

Figure 9.6   Case history 6: Nora's iris

banana, lemon juice, fish and lightly cooked vegetables. After
a few days she was able gradually to introduce normal foods
without producing symptoms.

Nora's stress levels were greatly reduced by taking vitamin B
complex with extra pantothenic acid, vitamins C and E, and
by having the opportunity to talk about her feelings to someone who was impartial.

Case History 7

Stephen, who is 40 years old, is a social worker. He came for
iris diagnosis because of possible food allergies. He
complained of feeling dizzy at odd times of the day, waking up
at a regular time during the night, periods of shaking and
trembling, and headaches. He was about to take on a promotion within his work and he was worried that he might not
be able to cope with the greater responsibility that it
entailed.

His iris revealed a genetic disposition towards metabolic
disorders and, more specifically, poor blood sugar control.
His resulting symptoms were those of hypoglycaemia (low

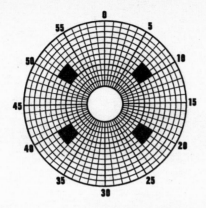

Figure 9.7   Case history 7: Stephen's iris

blood sugar). Further consultation showed that Stephen craved chocolate so much that he carried a couple of bars around with him in his car. He had become so worried that he was 'cracking up' but we were able to reassure him that there was nothing too seriously wrong. By restructuring his diet, adding supplements of vitamin B complex, vitamin C and zinc all his symptoms disappeared.

Case History 8

Vera, a sprightly 67 year old lady came for iris diagnosis because she was worried about her health generally and had arthritis in her hands. She was a very tense lady and was at her wits end because her husband was rapidly going deaf. The poor man would not go to his doctor, or do anything about it himself. This left Vera feeling very frustrated with him. Her mixed coloured iris revealed nothing untoward and we were able to reassure her.

Her arthritis was caused by her body retaining too much uric acid. This could be identified by the peculiar overlaid grey tones of her iris. Her adrenal showed a slight depletion

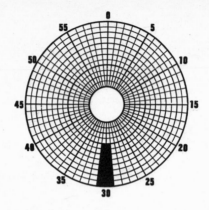

Figure 9.8   Case history 8: Vera's iris

which would be made up by her taking extra B vitamins. Calming and soothing herbs such as camomile, balm, valerian and scullcap were prescribed. To support her kidneys and aid the elimination of excess uric acid, gravel root and couch grass were given. After one month she reported a vast improvement of her symptoms, but not her husband's!

Case History 9

Mr X, a well known television personality, was examined at the television studio. He felt very well and claimed never to have had a day's illness in his life. Although he was rather over-weight, he said it did not interfere with his health. As the moment drew near when he was to make his 'live' appearance, the atmosphere in the studio was electric, nerves became tense and everyone looked anxious. Little beads of perspiration appeared on Mr X's forehead but he said he felt quite calm.

His iris was extremely clear and free from genetic markings except for one which appeared in his heart zone. We urged Mr X to seek further advice from his doctor and to reduce his

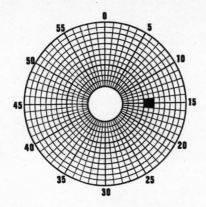

Figure 9.9 Case history 9: Mr X's iris

weight seriously. Eighteen months later Mr X sadly died suddenly from a heart attack.

Case History 10

A young girl, six year old Bobby, was brought by her worried mother. The child had periods of irritability and depression, together with abdominal pain, especially around the umbilicus, with periods of diarrhoea. There was discourse in the family home as she seemed unable to eat a proper meal – this caused her father much irritation and concern. Bobby was not a happy child, despite the fact that she was well cared for.

Her iris at once revealed the trouble. When asked, her mother confirmed that Bobby was 'a nose picker' and 'bottom scratcher'. This was confirmation of the iris signs for lower intestinal parasites, or worms. These kind of infestations are quite common, particularly in children of Bobby's age. However, by applying some very simple measures, such unwanted guests can be eradicated. Tansy is the herb we find successful for ridding the body of worms. This should then be followed up by a good bowel tonic such as camomile, balm,

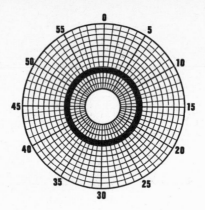

Figure 9.10   Case history 10: Bobby's iris

barberry and slippery elm. Within a few days Bobby was full of
life, happier and eating better-sized meals.

Case History 11

Rose, a social worker, came to see us because she felt generally
unwell and wondered if iridology could provide the answers
which she had been seeking for some time. She was rather
overweight and was tired and irritable most of the time.

Her iris was blue, a weak connective tissue type and of the
lymphatic constitution. At 36 in her right iris (the gallbladder
zone) were a series of small black dots (defects). At 39 in her
right iris (the pancreas zone) were signs of inflammation.
These two signs were significant. Finally, there were signs of
weakness to the rectum zone. Her digestion was too slow and
she was able to open her bowels only every three or four
days.

We suggested further investigations should be made by the
hospital but, before the appointment was reached, she was
taken into hospital with severe abdominal pains. This was discovered as being pancreatitis (inflammation of the pancreas).

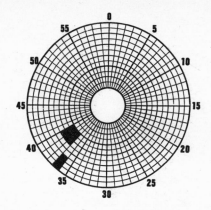

Figure 9.11   Case history 11: Rose's iris

Eventually, at a much later date, she had X-rays taken of her gallbladder. They revealed exactly what we had suspected: there were 8 to 10 large stones. We decided that, in view of the size of the stones, an operation would be the best way for her to regain her health. We therefore prescribed a course of vitamins and minerals to help build up her body in readiness for the operation.

Case History 12

Wendy, a housewife, came to see us because she wanted to lose weight. She was about 14 kg over her 'normal' weight and had tried everything to reduce but without success. She assured us that she did not eat excessively although she did admit to the odd craving for chocolate. Wendy had tried many different types of popular diets – all to no avail. She simply could not understand why her weight would not reduce. Tiredness, exhaustion and indigestion were among her symptoms.

We often find that the cause of being overweight is not just simply the *amount* of food but it is the type which is important.

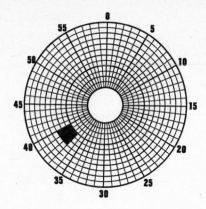

. *Figure 9.12*   Case history 12: Wendy's iris

Not only that, it rather depends what your body does, or does not do, with the food once it has been eaten. The glands of the body affect metabolism and therefore weight. Iridology is therefore a good way to check out the endocrine system which may be the first step in finding out *why* there is a weight problem. Incidentally, the same criteria apply if you are underweight.

Wendy's iris was of the mixed constitutional type (biliary). It showed the classic pre-diabetes pigmentations and an asthenic ridge running right through the pancreas zone. This was a sure indication that her pancreas was not functioning as well as it should, though, she could recall no family member who was a diabetic. Our diagnosis was hypoglycaemia - low blood sugar. We felt quite sure this was contributing to her weight problem.

We prescribed vitamin C 2mg, B complex, vitamin E 600 iu's, calcium pantothenic 100mg, a multimineral complex containing zinc and chromium and, finally, *lacto acidophilus*, the friendly bacteria. However by far the most important factor was diet which was restricted to small, regular meals containing balanced amounts of carbohydrate, fat and protein with absolutely no sugar – this was totally forbidden.

Wendy returned three months later overjoyed at having lost 10 kg in weight and feeling terrific!

Of course not *all* obesity is due to the same factors as Wendy's. There are many aspects of total health which must be considered before effective and lasting weight loss can be achieved.

10

The Golden Rules in Finding an Iridologist

The first golden rule in the search for an iridologist is for you to find him, and not for him to find you. There can be no better way than to be personally recommended by someone who has already consulted a particular iridologist. A good iridologist will have a good reputation as his reference. Most patients find their iridologist in this way.

The second golden rule is never make an appointment with an iridologist who advertises for, if he has put the name to advertising, he most certainly has not been trained by one of the established schools. Second to being personally recommended or being referred by your practitioner, the next best way is to write (with a stamped addressed envelope) to one of the established training colleges listed asking for a list of registered practitioners.

The third golden rule is to find out if the practitioner you have in mind is ethically guided and whether he works from a Code of Ethics laid down by a reputable training college. As a patient, you must have the means to complain and iron out any misunderstandings should the need arise. Unlikely as it may be, a practitioner who is found guilty of malpractice would have his name removed from the register.

In Great Britain there are at present no laws governing practitioners in alternative/complementary medicine. There is therefore nothing to stop any unqualified person calling himself an iridologist. It is, then, essential that those who are involved in training iridologists should establish the very highest standards. At the moment 1,000 hours' study (which combines theory and practical work) is deemed the minimum in the UK. The theory, which is usually based on correspondence and written study units, is supported by audio and video programmes. The practical application is supported by tutorials and seminars. The new graduate has the support of his college tutor for the first twelve months of his practice. The college is selective in who it trains and carefully assesses all would-be practitioners before they are allowed to practice. This differentiates its graduates from those who have studied for only 50 to 100 hours.

We have already stated that it is common for an iridologist to practise one of the healing arts (many homoeopaths are skilled iridologists) but beware the 'Jack of all Trades' for he is master of none. A string of meaningless letters after his name that is so long you could use it as a pole vault, often means he is a weekender, two days on a course and he knows it all!

Many well-meaning therapists have been tempted to add iridology to their list of skills and may have attended one of the popular two-day courses which spring up from time to time. However, we all know that real skill comes with a methodical and thorough knowledge of the subject which cannot be gained in a couple of days.

How Many Visits do I Have to Have?
Often only one or two visits are necessary. If the iridologist takes a photograph, a second visit is required if arrangements have been made for you to view your iris picture. If you are receiving treatment from your iridologist, there should be an improvement in your health within ten days; even the smallest of improvements should be viewed positively.

Does It Hurt?
No, iridology is completely safe and non-invasive. Occasionally

a patient may feel a little uncomfortable sitting close to the practitioner, or be unable to open their eye sufficiently for the iridologist to view the iris. In such a case the iridologist will probably take a picture without causing any further discomfort and ask you to return after a week to discuss the iris findings.

Will the Iridologist Refer Me to Another Practitioner?

The iridologist is well aware that one form of medicine does not exist which is a panacea for all ills. We are far too complex a being and, with our likes and dislikes, it is important to be guided in the right direction. The iridologist may refer you back to your family doctor for his help, though it may be necessary to refer you to an alternative/complementary practitioner who is more experienced in the particular treatment that you need. If spinal degeneration were suspected you would be referred to an osteopath or a chiropractor who will take an X-ray to observe precisely the degeneration occurring in the spine.

How Long Does the Consultation Last?

The consultation will last about one hour, although we have spent as long as two hours with some patients, for part of the iridologist's role – indeed, part of *any* practitioner's role – is to educate and teach patients to become self-reliant. This way, true health is achieved and the 'patient' stops being a patient dependent on a practitioner. This, of course, is not always easy. For many people, the visit to an iridologist is often their first encounter with alternative medicine and to have their habits of a lifetime reorganized is hard to take. It takes time and much compassion to explain the benefits of a wholefood diet, less meat, more fruit and so on.

Can Iridology Help Children?

This is a more difficult question. The ideal age for a child to see an iridologist is about six, for the iris is still forming up to this age. Taking a photograph of a very young child's eye is practically impossible. We have been photographing (or trying to) young children's eyes for many years and, out of ten photographs, only one would be of any use. It is far better for the iridologist to sit with the child close to a window so that the natural light illuminates the iris. This allows the iridologist a good look at the iris without causing the child any distress.

Useful Addresses

The National Council and Register of Iridologists
80 Portland Road
Bournemouth
BH9 1NQ
UK
(Telephone 0202 529793)
Professional organization offering training courses, seminars, iridology publications and video programmes. Iris photographic service. List of Registered Iridologists available.

Josef Angerer
Nederlinger Strasse 16
D-8000 Munchen 19
West Germany

Josef Angerer is one of the leading figures in iris diagnosis. His studies of the iris have been an inspiration to all those involved in this research.

Institute for Fundamental Research in Iris Diagnosis
D-7505
Ettlingen
West Germany

Joseph Deck runs training courses, but they are in German, although his books have been translated into English.

Iridology Research
35 Featherstone Street
London
EC1Y 8QX
UK
(Telephone 01 251 4429)

Iris photographic service available also supplier of books on Iridology and other related subjects.

National Iridology Research Association
POB 5277
Santa Fe
NM 87502
USA
(Telephone 505 983 6139)

American Association of Iridology, has books, tapes etc.

Dr Bernard Jensen
Route 1
Box 52
Escondido
California 92025
USA
(Telephone 714 749 2727)

Dr Jensen is perfecting a computer-assisted Iridology programme which we hope will soon be available.

Candida and Colon Clinic
93 Cheap Street
Sherborne
DT9 3LS
(Telephone 0935 813257)

Dr Harry Howell runs this centre for treatment of candidiasis and other fungal infections.

British School of Iridology
Dolphin House
6 Gold Stret
Saffron Walden
Essex
CB10 1EJ
UK
(Telephone 0799 26138)

Courses in Iridology which include personality readings from the iris.

The Institute for Complementary Medicine
21 Portland Place
London
W1N 3AF
UK
(Telephone 01 636 9543)

Publish a very usable reference book for all interested in Complementary Medicine. Holds an extensive list of reputable practitioners of all branches of Complementary Medicine.

School of Natural Healing
Thornham Herb garden
Thornham Magna,
Suffolk
UK
(Telephone 037 983 510)

Dr Kitty Campion and Dr Jill Davies in partnership run a wonderful herbal course based on the well-known teachings of the late Dr John Christopher.

National College of Holistic Medicine
26 Sea Road
Boscombe
Bournemouth
Dorset
UK
(Telephone 0202 36354)

Runs courses in colon cleansing and is also a residential health care centre.

Further Reading

Differentiation of Iris Markings, Josef Deck. An authoritative text book. Published by Institute for Fundamental Research in Iris Diagnosis, 1983. Available from Genesis Bookshop, 188 Old Street, London EC1 (01 250 1868).

Fundamental Basis of Iris Diagnosis, Theodor Kriege, L. N. Fowler, 1975.

Iridology: A Study of Health through the Iris, Dorothy Hall, Angus and Robertson, 1980.

Iridology Simplified, Bernard Jensen, Iridologists International, 1980. Available from Genesis Bookshop, 188 Old Street, London EC1 (01 250 1868).

Iridology Explained, James and Sheelagh Colton, J & S. Colton Health Publications, 1985. 80 Portland Road, Bournemouth BH9 1NQ (0202 529793).

Iris Diagnosis and Your Health, James and Sheelagh Colton, J. & S. Colton Health Publications, 1985. 80 Portland Road, Bournemouth BH9 1NQ (0202 529793).

The Institute for Complementary Medicine, Yearbook, W. Foulsham.

Index